HI!

Bet you didn't expect this.. I like to keep you on your toes.

I hope this journal will change your life.

Let's get going...

WELCOME TO YOUR JOURNAL!

First of all, well done for committing to bettering yourself.

Remember:
You will get out of this process what you put in.
Much like life in general!

This journal is to help guide you through the next 6 weeks of self improvement. Journalling helps you make sense of your thoughts & feelings, work through your limiting beliefs and stay accountable to your goals.

It's the cheapest therapy available!

At Commit to 6 our golden rule is to reach out if you need some support.

We are as committed to your goals as you are.

Commit to 6 team x

Journal number:

Name:

Date:

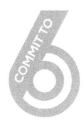

Section 1: Values

This section will help you identify your values. Put simply these are the things that are most important to you.

Knowing your values is important. It's the first step to living a life in line with what you believe in.

Your values should act like a compass guiding your decisions. Many of us let life happen to us and wonder through life without realising we aren't living it the way we had intended to. This journal will help you avoid that.

One of the reasons people struggle to meet their goals or find that they know what to do but aren't taking the action required is because their goals have not been set in line with their values. This is why we start with identifying your values

Once you have figured out what your values are and set your goals to align with these life becomes far more purposeful and fulfilling.

This is the key to living a life you love.

We recommend you identify a max of 4 values.

A list of values to help you pick:

Authenticity
Achievement
Adventure
Authority
Autonomy
Balance
Boldness
Compassion
Challenge
Community
Competency
Contribution
Creativity
Curiosity
Determination
Fairness
Faith
Fame

Friendships
Fun
Growth
Popularity
Recognition
Reputation
Respect
Responsibility
Security
Self-Respect
Service
Spirituality
Stability
Success
Status
Trustworthiness
Wealth
Wisdom

Health
Happiness
Honesty
Humor
Influence
Inner Harmony
Justice
Kindness
Knowledge
Leadership
Learning
Love
Loyalty
Openness
Optimism
Peace
Pleasure
Meaningful Work

Values are the underlying foundations of meaningful and fulfilling goals.

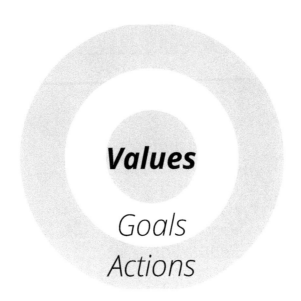

Identify your **top 3-4** *values:*

Now break these down into goals and then actions/habits in the next pages.

Example:

Value:

Health

Goals related to this value:

Fat loss

Increase activity

Exercise more

Action steps to reach your goal(s):

Stick to my weekly calorie
and step targets
A minimum of 3 workouts a week

Value:

Goals related to this value:

Action steps to reach your goal(s):

Value:

Goals related to this value:

Action steps to reach your goal(s):

Value:

Goals related to this value:

Action steps to reach your goal(s):

Value:

Goals related to this value:

Action steps to reach your goal(s):

Great, now you know your values...

Let's move on to section 2:

Taking action

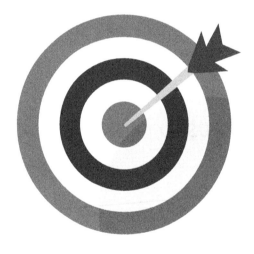

*Follow the rest of the journal & reflect
daily for the best results*

Quote of the week:

The aim isn't perfection.

Aiming for perfection is the easy option because it gives you the opportunity to quit if it can't be perfect.

Imperfect action takes that option away.

Intentions for the week:

How you want to show up

We all probably have an idea of how we want to show up, how we want to come across, the energy and VIBES we want to bring to life.

The best way to make sure you are creating the vibes you want is to be intentional with it.

I like to limit myself to 3 words.

Mine most weeks are:

Empowering
Engaging
Interested

3 must do's this week:
The 3 most important things I need to get done this week:

*Remember the aim is always to **under promise & over deliver**. This is a promise to yourself - don't break your own trust!*
*Note down **when** these should happen & **where** - this helps bridge the gap between intention and action.*

Keeping this to 3 will force you to prioritise.

Figure out what is most important based on your goals and values and focus on those tasks.

Delegate or delete the rest.

You probably don't need more time, you need more focus.

This kind of thinking will help you identify where you are wasting a lot of precious time doing things you don't need to do.

Mine this week:

Finish this journal (deadline TODAY)
Get back into a routine with exercise (5 gym sessions)
Book flights with Emilia

Date:

Today's Reflections:
What did I achieve today? what could I have done better? what did I learn? What negative thoughts did I have today? How can I reframe these into positives? **did I live in line with my values?**

Noting down daily wins helps you appreciate your progress – instead of waiting for the delayed reward you are focusing on winning each day.

Most days bring us some lessons too. You may not always act in line with your values – this isn't about beating yourself up if you don't. It's about learning from it so you can deal with it better next time. Remember we are here to help this too – if you need some help reach out in the group!

Leaning into negative emotions can teach you a lot about yourself. Instead of shutting them out try to figure out why you feel that way.

The most important question for me every day is did I live in line with my values. I don't nail it every day. But I learn when I don't.

If you want to live a fulfilling life that you love then I strongly recommend asking yourself this daily + being accountable to your actions.

Daily Accountability:

1) Activity
(Steps)

Write in your steps for the day

2) Nutrition
(Calories, protein, F&V)

Write in your nutrition stats for the day

3) Exercise
(Workout or rest day)

Write in your workout (or rest)

4) Mood & energy
(rate your mood & energy 1-10)

Check in with your mood/energy

Plan tomorrow:
What can you learn from today to make tomorrow better?
One thing you are going to do tomorrow for your future self.

This might be: same again – if you have had a great day or there may be some lessons.

The best days start with some planning. Don't hope things will fall into place. Make a plan and action them.

Making a plan is setting yourself up for success.

Weekly Review:

3 positives this week:

Celebrate your damn wins!
We tend to be EXCELLENT at identifying our failures but never giving ourselves credit for what we do well.
This could be things you are proud of or simply things that made you happy

3 lessons this week:

Negatives are great because we can learn from them. How's that for a reframe!.

3 things I am grateful for:

Bonus: if it's a person then reach out and tell them! You will make their day.

If every week was like this week would your future self be grateful?

If not, what do you need to work on next week?

This section is about owning your actions.

If you aren't living the life you want at the moment, what needs to change?

And whats one thing you can do this week to move you in the direction you want to go?

You won't change your life in 1 week but you can start!

That is quite enough from me - now it's your turn. The rest of the journal is for you to fill out. You will get the best results by committing to doing this EVERYDAY, without fail. ESPECIALLY on the days you don't want to do it.

Without exaggerating... doing this will change your life.

EG x

WEEK 1:

Quote of the week:

The aim isn't perfection.

Aiming for perfection is the easy option because it gives you the opportunity to quit if it can't be perfect.

Imperfect action takes that option away.

Intentions for the week:
How you want to show up

3 must do's this week:

The 3 most important things you need to get done this week:
*Remember the aim is always to **under promise & over deliver**. This is a promise to yourself - don't break your own trust!*
*Note down **when** these should happen & **where** - this helps bridge the gap between intention and action.*

Date:

Today's Reflections:

What did I achieve today? what could I have done better? what did I learn? What negative thoughts did I have today? How can I reframe these into positives? **did I live in line with my values?**

Daily Accountability:

1) Activity
(Steps)

2) Nutrition
(Calories, protein, F&V)

3) Exercise
(Workout or rest day)

4) Mood & energy
(rate your mood & energy 1-10)

Plan tomorrow:
What can you learn from today to make tomorrow better? Are there any negatives you can reframe into positives?
One thing you are going to do tomorrow for your future self.

Date:

Today's Reflections:

What did I achieve today? what could I have done better? what did I learn? What negative thoughts did I have today? How can I reframe these into positives? **did I live in line with my values?**

Daily Accountability:

1) Activity
(Steps)

2) Nutrition
(Calories, protein, F&V)

3) Exercise
(Workout or rest day)

4) Mood & energy
(rate your mood & energy 1-10)

Plan tomorrow:
What can you learn from today to make tomorrow better? Are there any negatives you can reframe into positives?
One thing you are going to do tomorrow for your future self.

Date:

Today's Reflections:

What did I achieve today? what could I have done better? what did I learn? What negative thoughts did I have today? How can I reframe these into positives? ***did I live in line with my values?***

Daily Accountability:

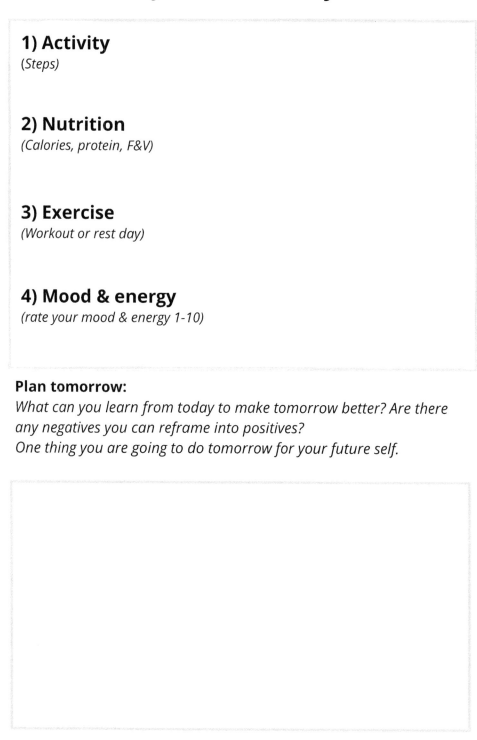

1) Activity
(Steps)

2) Nutrition
(Calories, protein, F&V)

3) Exercise
(Workout or rest day)

4) Mood & energy
(rate your mood & energy 1-10)

Plan tomorrow:
What can you learn from today to make tomorrow better? Are there any negatives you can reframe into positives?
One thing you are going to do tomorrow for your future self.

Date:

Today's Reflections:
What did I achieve today? what could I have done better? what did I learn? What negative thoughts did I have today? How can I reframe these into positives? **did I live in line with my values?**

Daily Accountability:

1) Activity
(Steps)

2) Nutrition
(Calories, protein, F&V)

3) Exercise
(Workout or rest day)

4) Mood & energy
(rate your mood & energy 1-10)

Plan tomorrow:
What can you learn from today to make tomorrow better? Are there any negatives you can reframe into positives?
One thing you are going to do tomorrow for your future self.

Date:

Today's Reflections:

What did I achieve today? what could I have done better? what did I learn? What negative thoughts did I have today? How can I reframe these into positives? **did I live in line with my values?**

Daily Accountability:

1) Activity
(Steps)

2) Nutrition
(Calories, protein, F&V)

3) Exercise
(Workout or rest day)

4) Mood & energy
(rate your mood & energy 1-10)

Plan tomorrow:
What can you learn from today to make tomorrow better? Are there any negatives you can reframe into positives?
One thing you are going to do tomorrow for your future self.

Date:

Today's Reflections:

What did I achieve today? what could I have done better? what did I learn? What negative thoughts did I have today? How can I reframe these into positives? ***did I live in line with my values?***

Daily Accountability:

1) Activity
(Steps)

2) Nutrition
(Calories, protein, F&V)

3) Exercise
(Workout or rest day)

4) Mood & energy
(rate your mood & energy 1-10)

Plan tomorrow:
What can you learn from today to make tomorrow better? Are there any negatives you can reframe into positives?
One thing you are going to do tomorrow for your future self.

Date:

Today's Reflections:

What did I achieve today? what could I have done better? what did I learn? What negative thoughts did I have today? How can I reframe these into positives? ***did I live in line with my values?***

Daily Accountability:

1) Activity
(Steps)

2) Nutrition
(Calories, protein, F&V)

3) Exercise
(Workout or rest day)

4) Mood & energy
(rate your mood & energy 1-10)

Plan tomorrow:

What can you learn from today to make tomorrow better? Are there any negatives you can reframe into positives?
One thing you are going to do tomorrow for your future self.

Weekly Review:

3 positives this week:

3 lessons this week:

3 things I am grateful for:

If every week was like this week would your future self be grateful?

If not, what do you need to work on next week?

If it has been a tough week remember that those are the weeks you learn from the most!

WEEK 2:

Quote of the week:

You get out what you put in.

Don't complain about the results you didn't get from the work you didn't do.

Intentions for the week:

How you want to show up

3 must do's this week:

The 3 most important things you need to get done this week:
*Remember the aim is always to **under promise & over deliver**. This is a promise to yourself - don't break your own trust!*
*Note down **when** these should happen & **where** - this helps bridge the gap between intention and action.*

Date:

Today's Reflections:
What did I achieve today? what could I have done better? what did I learn? What negative thoughts did I have today? How can I reframe these into positives? **did I live in line with my values?**

Daily Accountability:

1) Activity
(Steps)

2) Nutrition
(Calories, protein, F&V)

3) Exercise
(Workout or rest day)

4) Mood & energy
(rate your mood & energy 1-10)

Plan tomorrow:

What can you learn from today to make tomorrow better? Are there any negatives you can reframe into positives?
One thing you are going to do tomorrow for your future self.

Date:

Today's Reflections:

What did I achieve today? what could I have done better? what did I learn? What negative thoughts did I have today? How can I reframe these into positives? **did I live in line with my values?**

Daily Accountability:

1) Activity
(Steps)

2) Nutrition
(Calories, protein, F&V)

3) Exercise
(Workout or rest day)

4) Mood & energy
(rate your mood & energy 1-10)

Plan tomorrow:

What can you learn from today to make tomorrow better? Are there any negatives you can reframe into positives?
One thing you are going to do tomorrow for your future self.

Date:

Today's Reflections:

What did I achieve today? what could I have done better? what did I learn? What negative thoughts did I have today? How can I reframe these into positives? ***did I live in line with my values?***

Daily Accountability:

1) Activity
(Steps)

2) Nutrition
(Calories, protein, F&V)

3) Exercise
(Workout or rest day)

4) Mood & energy
(rate your mood & energy 1-10)

Plan tomorrow:
What can you learn from today to make tomorrow better? Are there any negatives you can reframe into positives?
One thing you are going to do tomorrow for your future self.

Date:

Today's Reflections:

What did I achieve today? what could I have done better? what did I learn? What negative thoughts did I have today? How can I reframe these into positives? **did I live in line with my values?**

Daily Accountability:

1) Activity
(Steps)

2) Nutrition
(Calories, protein, F&V)

3) Exercise
(Workout or rest day)

4) Mood & energy
(rate your mood & energy 1-10)

Plan tomorrow:
What can you learn from today to make tomorrow better? Are there any negatives you can reframe into positives?
One thing you are going to do tomorrow for your future self.

Date:

Today's Reflections:

What did I achieve today? what could I have done better? what did I learn? What negative thoughts did I have today? How can I reframe these into positives? ***did I live in line with my values?***

Daily Accountability:

1) Activity
(Steps)

2) Nutrition
(Calories, protein, F&V)

3) Exercise
(Workout or rest day)

4) Mood & energy
(rate your mood & energy 1-10)

Plan tomorrow:
What can you learn from today to make tomorrow better? Are there any negatives you can reframe into positives?
One thing you are going to do tomorrow for your future self.

Date:

Today's Reflections:

What did I achieve today? what could I have done better? what did I learn? What negative thoughts did I have today? How can I reframe these into positives? **did I live in line with my values?**

Daily Accountability:

1) Activity
(Steps)

2) Nutrition
(Calories, protein, F&V)

3) Exercise
(Workout or rest day)

4) Mood & energy
(rate your mood & energy 1-10)

Plan tomorrow:
What can you learn from today to make tomorrow better? Are there any negatives you can reframe into positives?
One thing you are going to do tomorrow for your future self.

Date:

Today's Reflections:

What did I achieve today? what could I have done better? what did I learn? What negative thoughts did I have today? How can I reframe these into positives? **did I live in line with my values?**

Daily Accountability:

1) Activity
(Steps)

2) Nutrition
(Calories, protein, F&V)

3) Exercise
(Workout or rest day)

4) Mood & energy
(rate your mood & energy 1-10)

Plan tomorrow:
What can you learn from today to make tomorrow better? Are there any negatives you can reframe into positives?
One thing you are going to do tomorrow for your future self.

Weekly Review:

3 positives this week:

3 lessons this week:

3 things I am grateful for:

If every week was like this week would your future self be grateful?

If not, what do you need to work on next week?

If it has been a tough week remember that those are the weeks you learn from the most!

Quote of the week:

The secret to success is not giving up.

The most common reason people don't achieve their goals is that they give up too soon

Intentions for the week:

How you want to show up

3 must do's this week:

The 3 most important things you need to get done this week:
*Remember the aim is always to **under promise & over deliver**. This is a promise to yourself - don't break your own trust!*
*Note down **when** these should happen & **where** - this helps bridge the gap between intention and action.*

Date:

Today's Reflections:

What did I achieve today? what could I have done better? what did I learn? What negative thoughts did I have today? How can I reframe these into positives? ***did I live in line with my values?***

Daily Accountability:

1) Activity
(Steps)

2) Nutrition
(Calories, protein, F&V)

3) Exercise
(Workout or rest day)

4) Mood & energy
(rate your mood & energy 1-10)

Plan tomorrow:
What can you learn from today to make tomorrow better? Are there any negatives you can reframe into positives?
One thing you are going to do tomorrow for your future self.

Date:

Today's Reflections:

What did I achieve today? what could I have done better? what did I learn? What negative thoughts did I have today? How can I reframe these into positives? **did I live in line with my values?**

Daily Accountability:

1) Activity
(Steps)

2) Nutrition
(Calories, protein, F&V)

3) Exercise
(Workout or rest day)

4) Mood & energy
(rate your mood & energy 1-10)

Plan tomorrow:
What can you learn from today to make tomorrow better? Are there any negatives you can reframe into positives?
One thing you are going to do tomorrow for your future self.

Date:

Today's Reflections:

What did I achieve today? what could I have done better? what did I learn? What negative thoughts did I have today? How can I reframe these into positives? **did I live in line with my values?**

Daily Accountability:

1) Activity
(Steps)

2) Nutrition
(Calories, protein, F&V)

3) Exercise
(Workout or rest day)

4) Mood & energy
(rate your mood & energy 1-10)

Plan tomorrow:
What can you learn from today to make tomorrow better? Are there any negatives you can reframe into positives?
One thing you are going to do tomorrow for your future self.

Date:

Today's Reflections:

What did I achieve today? what could I have done better? what did I learn? What negative thoughts did I have today? How can I reframe these into positives? **did I live in line with my values?**

Daily Accountability:

1) Activity
(Steps)

2) Nutrition
(Calories, protein, F&V)

3) Exercise
(Workout or rest day)

4) Mood & energy
(rate your mood & energy 1-10)

Plan tomorrow:
What can you learn from today to make tomorrow better? Are there any negatives you can reframe into positives?
One thing you are going to do tomorrow for your future self.

Date:

Today's Reflections:

What did I achieve today? what could I have done better? what did I learn? What negative thoughts did I have today? How can I reframe these into positives? **did I live in line with my values?**

Daily Accountability:

1) Activity
(Steps)

2) Nutrition
(Calories, protein, F&V)

3) Exercise
(Workout or rest day)

4) Mood & energy
(rate your mood & energy 1-10)

Plan tomorrow:
What can you learn from today to make tomorrow better? Are there any negatives you can reframe into positives?
One thing you are going to do tomorrow for your future self.

Date:

Today's Reflections:

What did I achieve today? what could I have done better? what did I learn? What negative thoughts did I have today? How can I reframe these into positives? ***did I live in line with my values?***

Daily Accountability:

1) Activity
(Steps)

2) Nutrition
(Calories, protein, F&V)

3) Exercise
(Workout or rest day)

4) Mood & energy
(rate your mood & energy 1-10)

Plan tomorrow:
What can you learn from today to make tomorrow better? Are there any negatives you can reframe into positives?
One thing you are going to do tomorrow for your future self.

Date:

Today's Reflections:
What did I achieve today? what could I have done better? what did I learn? What negative thoughts did I have today? How can I reframe these into positives? **did I live in line with my values?**

Daily Accountability:

1) Activity
(Steps)

2) Nutrition
(Calories, protein, F&V)

3) Exercise
(Workout or rest day)

4) Mood & energy
(rate your mood & energy 1-10)

Plan tomorrow:
What can you learn from today to make tomorrow better? Are there any negatives you can reframe into positives?
One thing you are going to do tomorrow for your future self.

Weekly Review:

3 positives this week:

3 lessons this week:

3 things I am grateful for:

If every week was like this week would your future self be grateful?

If not, what do you need to work on next week?

If it has been a tough week remember that those are the weeks you learn from the most!

Quote of the week:

Your future depends on the choices you make today.

They may seem insignificant now but your future self will thank you for them

Intentions for the week:

How you want to show up

3 must do's this week:

The 3 most important things you need to get done this week:
*Remember the aim is always to **under promise & over deliver**. This is a promise to yourself - don't break your own trust!*
*Note down **when** these should happen & **where** - this helps bridge the gap between intention and action.*

Date:

Today's Reflections:
What did I achieve today? what could I have done better? what did I learn? What negative thoughts did I have today? How can I reframe these into positives? **did I live in line with my values?**

Daily Accountability:

1) Activity
(Steps)

2) Nutrition
(Calories, protein, F&V)

3) Exercise
(Workout or rest day)

4) Mood & energy
(rate your mood & energy 1-10)

Plan tomorrow:
What can you learn from today to make tomorrow better? Are there any negatives you can reframe into positives?
One thing you are going to do tomorrow for your future self.

Date:

Today's Reflections:

What did I achieve today? what could I have done better? what did I learn? What negative thoughts did I have today? How can I reframe these into positives? **did I live in line with my values?**

Daily Accountability:

1) Activity
(Steps)

2) Nutrition
(Calories, protein, F&V)

3) Exercise
(Workout or rest day)

4) Mood & energy
(rate your mood & energy 1-10)

Plan tomorrow:
What can you learn from today to make tomorrow better? Are there any negatives you can reframe into positives?
One thing you are going to do tomorrow for your future self.

Date:

Today's Reflections:

What did I achieve today? what could I have done better? what did I learn? What negative thoughts did I have today? How can I reframe these into positives? **did I live in line with my values?**

Daily Accountability:

1) Activity
(Steps)

2) Nutrition
(Calories, protein, F&V)

3) Exercise
(Workout or rest day)

4) Mood & energy
(rate your mood & energy 1-10)

Plan tomorrow:
What can you learn from today to make tomorrow better? Are there any negatives you can reframe into positives?
One thing you are going to do tomorrow for your future self.

Date:

Today's Reflections:

What did I achieve today? what could I have done better? what did I learn? What negative thoughts did I have today? How can I reframe these into positives? **did I live in line with my values?**

Daily Accountability:

1) Activity
(Steps)

2) Nutrition
(Calories, protein, F&V)

3) Exercise
(Workout or rest day)

4) Mood & energy
(rate your mood & energy 1-10)

Plan tomorrow:
What can you learn from today to make tomorrow better? Are there any negatives you can reframe into positives?
One thing you are going to do tomorrow for your future self.

Date:

Today's Reflections:

What did I achieve today? what could I have done better? what did I learn? What negative thoughts did I have today? How can I reframe these into positives? ***did I live in line with my values?***

Daily Accountability:

1) Activity
(Steps)

2) Nutrition
(Calories, protein, F&V)

3) Exercise
(Workout or rest day)

4) Mood & energy
(rate your mood & energy 1-10)

Plan tomorrow:
What can you learn from today to make tomorrow better? Are there any negatives you can reframe into positives?
One thing you are going to do tomorrow for your future self.

Date:

Today's Reflections:
What did I achieve today? what could I have done better? what did I learn? What negative thoughts did I have today? How can I reframe these into positives? **did I live in line with my values?**

Daily Accountability:

1) Activity
(Steps)

2) Nutrition
(Calories, protein, F&V)

3) Exercise
(Workout or rest day)

4) Mood & energy
(rate your mood & energy 1-10)

Plan tomorrow:
What can you learn from today to make tomorrow better? Are there any negatives you can reframe into positives?
One thing you are going to do tomorrow for your future self.

Date:

Today's Reflections:

What did I achieve today? what could I have done better? what did I learn? What negative thoughts did I have today? How can I reframe these into positives? **did I live in line with my values?**

Daily Accountability:

1) Activity
(Steps)

2) Nutrition
(Calories, protein, F&V)

3) Exercise
(Workout or rest day)

4) Mood & energy
(rate your mood & energy 1-10)

Plan tomorrow:
What can you learn from today to make tomorrow better? Are there any negatives you can reframe into positives?
One thing you are going to do tomorrow for your future self.

Weekly Review:

3 positives this week:

3 lessons this week:

3 things I am grateful for:

If every week was like this week would your future self be grateful?

If not, what do you need to work on next week?

If it has been a tough week remember that those are the weeks you learn from the most!

WEEK 5:

Quote of the week:

Motivation is a byproduct of action.
& lack of action feeds lack of motivation.

If you want to feel better you often have to take
the first step before you want to.

Intentions for the week:

How you want to show up

3 must do's this week:

The 3 most important things you need to get done this week:
*Remember the aim is always to **under promise & over deliver**. This is a promise to yourself - don't break your own trust!*
*Note down **when** these should happen & **where** - this helps bridge the gap between intention and action.*

Date:

Today's Reflections:
What did I achieve today? what could I have done better? what did I learn? What negative thoughts did I have today? How can I reframe these into positives? **did I live in line with my values?**

Daily Accountability:

1) Activity
(Steps)

2) Nutrition
(Calories, protein, F&V)

3) Exercise
(Workout or rest day)

4) Mood & energy
(rate your mood & energy 1-10)

Plan tomorrow:
What can you learn from today to make tomorrow better? Are there any negatives you can reframe into positives?
One thing you are going to do tomorrow for your future self.

Date:

Today's Reflections:

What did I achieve today? what could I have done better? what did I learn? What negative thoughts did I have today? How can I reframe these into positives? ***did I live in line with my values?***

Daily Accountability:

1) Activity
(Steps)

2) Nutrition
(Calories, protein, F&V)

3) Exercise
(Workout or rest day)

4) Mood & energy
(rate your mood & energy 1-10)

Plan tomorrow:
What can you learn from today to make tomorrow better? Are there any negatives you can reframe into positives?
One thing you are going to do tomorrow for your future self.

Date:

Today's Reflections:
What did I achieve today? what could I have done better? what did I learn? What negative thoughts did I have today? How can I reframe these into positives? **did I live in line with my values?**

Daily Accountability:

1) Activity
(Steps)

2) Nutrition
(Calories, protein, F&V)

3) Exercise
(Workout or rest day)

4) Mood & energy
(rate your mood & energy 1-10)

Plan tomorrow:
What can you learn from today to make tomorrow better? Are there any negatives you can reframe into positives?
One thing you are going to do tomorrow for your future self.

Date:

Today's Reflections:

What did I achieve today? what could I have done better? what did I learn? What negative thoughts did I have today? How can I reframe these into positives? **did I live in line with my values?**

Daily Accountability:

1) Activity
(Steps)

2) Nutrition
(Calories, protein, F&V)

3) Exercise
(Workout or rest day)

4) Mood & energy
(rate your mood & energy 1-10)

Plan tomorrow:
What can you learn from today to make tomorrow better? Are there any negatives you can reframe into positives?
One thing you are going to do tomorrow for your future self.

Date:

Today's Reflections:

What did I achieve today? what could I have done better? what did I learn? What negative thoughts did I have today? How can I reframe these into positives? ***did I live in line with my values?***

Daily Accountability:

1) Activity
(Steps)

2) Nutrition
(Calories, protein, F&V)

3) Exercise
(Workout or rest day)

4) Mood & energy
(rate your mood & energy 1-10)

Plan tomorrow:
What can you learn from today to make tomorrow better? Are there any negatives you can reframe into positives?
One thing you are going to do tomorrow for your future self.

Date:

Today's Reflections:

What did I achieve today? what could I have done better? what did I learn? What negative thoughts did I have today? How can I reframe these into positives? **did I live in line with my values?**

Daily Accountability:

1) Activity
(Steps)

2) Nutrition
(Calories, protein, F&V)

3) Exercise
(Workout or rest day)

4) Mood & energy
(rate your mood & energy 1-10)

Plan tomorrow:

What can you learn from today to make tomorrow better? Are there any negatives you can reframe into positives?
One thing you are going to do tomorrow for your future self.

Date:

Today's Reflections:
What did I achieve today? what could I have done better? what did I learn? What negative thoughts did I have today? How can I reframe these into positives? **did I live in line with my values?**

Daily Accountability:

1) Activity
(Steps)

2) Nutrition
(Calories, protein, F&V)

3) Exercise
(Workout or rest day)

4) Mood & energy
(rate your mood & energy 1-10)

Plan tomorrow:

What can you learn from today to make tomorrow better? Are there any negatives you can reframe into positives?
One thing you are going to do tomorrow for your future self.

Weekly Review:

3 positives this week:

3 lessons this week:

3 things I am grateful for:

If every week was like this week would your future self be grateful?
If not, what do you need to work on next week?

If it has been a tough week remember that those are the weeks you learn from the most!

Quitting won't speed up the process.

If you are living your life whilst working towards your goals, you'll need far less patience because you are no longer waiting for anything.

Intentions for the week:

How you want to show up

3 must do's this week:

The 3 most important things you need to get done this week:
*Remember the aim is always to **under promise & over deliver**. This is a promise to yourself - don't break your own trust!*
*Note down **when** these should happen & **where** - this helps bridge the gap between intention and action.*

Date:

Today's Reflections:
What did I achieve today? what could I have done better? what did I learn? What negative thoughts did I have today? How can I reframe these into positives? **did I live in line with my values?**

Daily Accountability:

1) Activity
(Steps)

2) Nutrition
(Calories, protein, F&V)

3) Exercise
(Workout or rest day)

4) Mood & energy
(rate your mood & energy 1-10)

Plan tomorrow:

What can you learn from today to make tomorrow better? Are there any negatives you can reframe into positives?
One thing you are going to do tomorrow for your future self.

Date:

Today's Reflections:

What did I achieve today? what could I have done better? what did I learn? What negative thoughts did I have today? How can I reframe these into positives? **did I live in line with my values?**

Daily Accountability:

1) Activity
(Steps)

2) Nutrition
(Calories, protein, F&V)

3) Exercise
(Workout or rest day)

4) Mood & energy
(rate your mood & energy 1-10)

Plan tomorrow:

What can you learn from today to make tomorrow better? Are there any negatives you can reframe into positives?
One thing you are going to do tomorrow for your future self.

Date:

Today's Reflections:
What did I achieve today? what could I have done better? what did I learn? What negative thoughts did I have today? How can I reframe these into positives? **did I live in line with my values?**

Daily Accountability:

1) Activity
(Steps)

2) Nutrition
(Calories, protein, F&V)

3) Exercise
(Workout or rest day)

4) Mood & energy
(rate your mood & energy 1-10)

Plan tomorrow:

What can you learn from today to make tomorrow better? Are there any negatives you can reframe into positives?
One thing you are going to do tomorrow for your future self.

Date:

Today's Reflections:

What did I achieve today? what could I have done better? what did I learn? What negative thoughts did I have today? How can I reframe these into positives? **did I live in line with my values?**

Daily Accountability:

1) Activity
(Steps)

2) Nutrition
(Calories, protein, F&V)

3) Exercise
(Workout or rest day)

4) Mood & energy
(rate your mood & energy 1-10)

Plan tomorrow:
What can you learn from today to make tomorrow better? Are there any negatives you can reframe into positives?
One thing you are going to do tomorrow for your future self.

Date:

Today's Reflections:
What did I achieve today? what could I have done better? what did I learn? What negative thoughts did I have today? How can I reframe these into positives? **did I live in line with my values?**

Daily Accountability:

1) Activity
(Steps)

2) Nutrition
(Calories, protein, F&V)

3) Exercise
(Workout or rest day)

4) Mood & energy
(rate your mood & energy 1-10)

Plan tomorrow:

What can you learn from today to make tomorrow better? Are there any negatives you can reframe into positives?
One thing you are going to do tomorrow for your future self.

Date:

Today's Reflections:
What did I achieve today? what could I have done better? what did I learn? What negative thoughts did I have today? How can I reframe these into positives? **did I live in line with my values?**

Daily Accountability:

1) Activity
(Steps)

2) Nutrition
(Calories, protein, F&V)

3) Exercise
(Workout or rest day)

4) Mood & energy
(rate your mood & energy 1-10)

Plan tomorrow:

What can you learn from today to make tomorrow better? Are there any negatives you can reframe into positives?
One thing you are going to do tomorrow for your future self.

Date:

Today's Reflections:

What did I achieve today? what could I have done better? what did I learn? What negative thoughts did I have today? How can I reframe these into positives? **did I live in line with my values?**

Daily Accountability:

1) Activity
(Steps)

2) Nutrition
(Calories, protein, F&V)

3) Exercise
(Workout or rest day)

4) Mood & energy
(rate your mood & energy 1-10)

Plan tomorrow:
What can you learn from today to make tomorrow better? Are there any negatives you can reframe into positives?
One thing you are going to do tomorrow for your future self.

Weekly Review:

3 positives this week:

3 lessons this week:

3 things I am grateful for:

If every week was like this week would your future self be grateful?

If not, what do you need to work on next week?

If it has been a tough week remember that those are the weeks you learn from the most!

6 week Review

3 things you've learnt over the last 6 weeks:

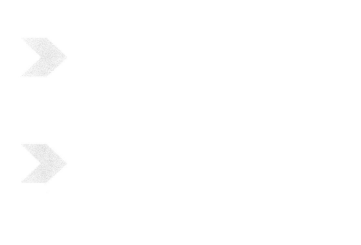

Space to review your last 6 weeks & what you can improve on going forward:

Give yourself a pat on the back because you should be proud of yourself for the effort you've put in over the last 6 weeks.

Don't forget to check in with your coach to review progress.

ESG x